THE INTELLIGENT NURSE ™

Nursing Skills for the 21st Century to Improve Patient Safety and Satisfaction

By Donald Wood, ARNP, CRNA

Intelligent:

displaying or characterized by quickness of understanding, sound thought, or good judgment

Nurse:

a licensed healthcare professional who practices independently or is supervised by a physician, surgeon, or dentist and who is skilled in promoting and maintaining health

The Intelligent Nurse ™:

a nurse who knows how to positively affect her/his patients, co-workers and organization through superior knowledge of communicating, planning, leadership, critical thinking and other 21st Century nursing skills.

Acknowledgements

My wife, Debbie, has been my number one supporter throughout the development of this book. Her comments and suggestions and have been invaluable. Besides, anyone who can put up with me for this many years is a saint!

Many thanks to Mr. Ed Greenberg, President of Hound Dog Hearing (www.hdhearing.com) of Washington, D.C., for allowing the use of figure 1. Hound Dog Hearing markets assistive listening devices for people who have hearing deficits.

Jessi Hoffman edited this book and gave me innumerable suggestions that were extremely valuable. My profound thanks to her for her great work.

CONTENTS

INTRODUCTION

Nursing care has traditionally been centered on the assessment of patients, providing for their needs and administering medication or treatments that have been prescribed. Since 1860 when Florence Nightingale opened the Nightingale Training School, progress in nursing has occurred in a slow, often spasmodic fashion. Throughout this time period, nursing was placed (somewhat contentedly) in a position that was subservient to physicians. If a physician entered the nurse's station, a nurse was obliged to stand up and let the physician have her seat. This pretty much described hospital nursing for many years.

In the late 1960s, some units started to advance in the technology of caring for higher-acuity patients. Consequently, the nurses in those units had more information to base their nursing diagnoses on and were able to react to changes in a patient's condition in a rapid fashion. These nurses in the early intensive and cardiac care units were often given a small amount of latitude for autonomy at the bedside.

A certain respect arose between such nurses and the physicians who worked in those units. Other than in those instances, it was still slow going for the basic bedside nurse where leadership was concerned. Consequently, she had little need for leadership skills. Thankfully, progress has occurred over the past four decades.

Nursing outside of the hospital has some differences depending on the actual type of nursing practice. Work in a medical office, insurance company, home health or other setting can involve specialized skill sets but still makes use of the basics taught in nursing school. If you made it through nursing school and were smart enough to obtain your nursing license, you can probably exist in a nursing job for years and just coast along. Mediocrity reigns, are you getting wet? Most nurses will obtain the continuing education units they are required to have in order to renew their nursing license, but will do little more. (Often their choice of classes is determined by which is the cheapest.) Some others will look at their basic nursing as a prelude to moving into advanced practice.

A nurse in the 21st Century is capable of much more than nurses of the past ever dreamed of. The nurse of today is a valued professional who is respected by the public more than people in any other profession (according to a recent Gallup Poll). Today's nurse can rise to the top level of management in any organization. The educational opportunities available, both formal and otherwise, are limited only by the desires of the individual. Advanced practice, business, and other career routes are available depending on the goals you may have.

The Intelligent Nurse Program seeks to lay a 21st Century foundation for every nurse. The subjects covered in this program are meant to enhance the everyday tasks that any nurse performs. These enhancements can be far-reaching and affect such things as patient safety, patient satisfaction, and your own job satisfaction. At the same time, we teach skills that are not traditionally thought of in the nursing realm.

Many nursing programs have a course on nursing leadership, but do these courses teach you to lead your patient? Do these courses teach you the fine points of being a good follower? How about leading those in a position above you? Leadership is usually taught as the work performed in a leadership or policy-making position (nurse manager, director, chief nursing officer). The truth of the matter is, you don't need a title or position to be a leader, and good leadership skills are often required of nurses at lower levels of an organization.

Leadership is especially critical now. We are in an era where a significant number of patient deaths and injuries are generated by preventable causes. It takes someone with more than a basic nursing education to know when and how to intervene to stop an accident from occurring. This requires the ability to keep details in focus while looking at the big picture. It calls for the aptitude of questioning a physician's decision when an inappropriate order is given. It demands the capacity to know how to do these things and still be seen as part of a cohesive, patient-focused team.

Being *The Intelligent Nurse* is not a hard thing to do. It is well within the capability of every nurse today to accomplish. Once this knowledge is gained and placed into use, others will notice the difference in you. You will become the "go-to" person on your unit, the nurse that patients send thank-you cards to.

COMMUNICATING

Communication is the exchange of information – often vital information – between two parties. This exchange can take place on many levels simultaneously. Excellent communication is extremely important to the provision of good patient care.

Every nurse is aware of the distinction between verbal and nonverbal communication. Tone of voice, vocal volume, facial expression, body posture, and hand gestures are but a few of the ways we communicate with others. Occasionally we send out mixed signals that become confusing. Telling someone they are doing a great job while rolling our eyes leaves the other person wondering what was truly meant. When the meaning of the message is open for interpretation, you can be sure the correct message has a slim chance of getting across.

Add to that the fact that we use many terms in a way that is contrary to what we are saying. How many medical people have asked a patient if they want a pain shot? The correct way to get the desired information would be to ask if the patient is in pain and then offer an appropriate analgesic or pain relief medication. Precision in communication is mandatory.

I once had a young female patient who spoke only Spanish. She was scheduled for emergency surgery late one evening. None of the members of the call team with me in the operating room could speak Spanish. We can often bridge a communication gap by way of pictures, hand gestures, and so on (nonverbal communication) when the patient is awake and alert. My concern centered on the ability to communicate with this woman as she was emerging from anesthesia. This is a time when it is extremely difficult to decipher nonverbal communications. It was essential to have a means of communicating with her verbally. I boiled my requirements down to the basics. I needed to know how to say "Wake up," "Take a deep breath," and "Are you in pain?"

Luckily for me, one of the nurses on the surgical floor spoke Spanish. I sought her out and told her of my needs. A very brief language lesson ensued in the hallway. During that time, I became conversant in the three phrases I would need to communicate with the patient during a time that is confusing to people even when there is no language barrier.

This small step allowed me to tell the patient that her procedure was finished, encourage deep breathing, and assess her need for analgesic medication in the immediate post-operative period. Through the appropriate use of available resources and my new-found communication skill, I was The Intelligent Nurse.

Communication Essentials

Many definitions of the word "communication" stress the passing of information from one point to another. But effective communication includes more than that. It requires that the information sender confirm that the recipient actually received *and* understood the information. This is a matter of determining whether "what I think I said is what you think you heard."

Many industries that depend on precise communication take steps to confirm that the information was transferred intact. When computers talk to each other, they typically have a built-in check against their original message. This is called a checksum. Basically, after a computer message is sent (via a series of ones and zeros), the final piece of information is mathematically based on the other sent information. If any of the information is missing or corrupt, the receiving computer will not be able to validate the checksum it receives. At that point, it requests an automatic re-transmission of the information. This is all based on the very precise language all computers utilize. No translation, no confusion.

A quick look at the aviation industry serves as another example of good communication. When the pilot of an aircraft receives a clearance for his flight from the air traffic controller, he must read back certain essential parts of the clearance.

Ground control: "*Cessna 2846* is cleared to the *Orlando Municipal* Airport *as filed*, climb and maintain *4,000* feet, departure control frequency *118.175*, squawk

[16]

0522." (The italicized areas indicate the essential items of this clearance.)

The pilot knows he will receive the information in a precise format consisting of the aircraft identification (Cessna 2846), clearance limit (Orlando Municipal), altitude to climb to (4,000 feet), radio frequency (118.175), and transponder setting (0522, referred to as "squawk"). The pilot will then respond (in the same order as received) as follows: "Cessna 2846, Orlando Municipal, 4,000, 118.175, 0522."

This tells the air traffic controller that the pilot received, heard, and understands the important parts of the clearance. If the information read back is correct, a quick "read-back correct" is given to the pilot to let him know his information is accurate. If the air traffic controller hears something on the read-back that doesn't agree with what he issued to the pilot, the errant piece of information is repeated and the discrepancy cleared up. Not until the pilot hears "read-back correct" does he know his understanding of the information is faultless.

So much care is given to accurate communication in the aviation industry in order to avoid life-threatening errors. Doesn't it make sense to pay equally close attention to accurate communication with our patients, since life-threatening mistakes also occur in the medical field?

Age-Related Issues

As time marches on, each new generation develops a mini-language of its own. The vocabulary may relate to certain segments of the culture (music or sports, for example) or may be more general terms that develop and take hold. While the meanings are well known to members of that generation, they often create confusing situations for people of other generations, leading to misunderstandings.

An example of such an age-related term is the word "bad." The online dictionary at www.dictionary.com lists 48 uses of this word. Forty-seven of those have a negative connotation. One usage of the word, the slang meaning, is "outstandingly excellent; first-rate." It doesn't take too much imagination to think of examples where a young, hip caregiver talking to an elderly patient could cause some confusion!

Other examples of slang use are sure to pop up in our daily conversations. We must take steps to ensure that our words come across to our patients as we intend. I read a book recently by Frank Luntz , titled *It's Not What You Say, It's What People Hear*. While primarily directed at the political scene, his message is equally applicable to healthcare. While our use of some terms might seem perfectly normal to us, we must be aware of the meaning that the person listening might give to our words.

Interestingly enough, the word "bad" actually had a good meaning behind it in the late 1890s. Maybe the new hip way to talk isn't so new after all!

Culture-Related Issues

Differences in culture commonly lead to difficulty in communications. The cultural differences may stem from differences in the country each of us was raised in or from different cultural subsets within the same country.

I once worked with three nurses from the Philippines, where there are two official languages: Filipino (Tagalog) and English. In addition, there are approximately 170 other languages, most stemming from various provinces within the country. Two of the nurses would frequently speak in a provincial language they knew but that the third nurse could not understand. When this happened you would hear the third nurse say (in English), "in Tagalog, in Tagalog."

In 1975, I moved from Florida to Columbia, South Carolina. I experienced a distinct culture shock that took many forms. In addition to the Blue Laws that were on the books in that state (you could purchase only food and medication there on Sundays), I found many words and sayings that were quite new to me.

On interviewing a patient before surgery, I asked if he had ever had any previous surgery. The patient told me he had once had a "bible bump" removed. I had absolutely no idea what he meant. I inquired a little further and found out that a bible bump refers to a ganglion cyst in the area of the wrist. The story goes that in days of old, the treatment for a ganglion cyst (which manifests itself as a tender raised area on the wrist) was to place the patient's wrist on a table and drop the heavy family Bible on the bump. The cyst would rupture, only to return in six to eight months. The term "bible bump" was used widely among long-term residents of South Carolina.

This was one of many communication stories that evolved during my two years in anesthesia school. Several students were from foreign countries, and we often had interesting conversations about our differences – speech being one of the more obvious.

If cultural differences pose communication problems, imagine the difficulties for a patient from another culture, with limited understanding of English, trying to relate to a caregiver who speaks in the technical language we call medicine! This is a job for The Intelligent Nurse! When in a situation like this, look at the patient's face. Often this observation is telling. When you see the head tilt, the forehead furrow, and other similar signs, you need to stop and assess the situation. Be sure the message you transmitted was received intact!

[21]

This is the time to ask the patient to repeat your explanation in his or her own words. Try to see what their understanding of your conversation was. It may require that you think of new words or use analogies to get your message across. If there are family members in the room, especially younger ones who have a better grasp of English, you may need to use them to help the process along. Another excellent choice is a certified interpreter.

Cultural miscommunication may also occur when one term has different meanings within two different cultures. It doesn't take a large language gap for something like this to occur. Words spoken by the British, although commonly used in the States, may have a different meaning here that causes some strange looks when uttered. The British term "cracking," for instance, has nothing to do with something about to break. It just means something is the best. When you are in England and someone asks if they can "knock you up," they mean may they knock on your door to awaken you. Then there is that awkward expression the Brits use in place of our "by golly": surprised Brits say, "Blow me"!

Hearing and Sight Impairment Issues

As some people age, their hearing reveals the stress and abuse of their earlier years. This abuse could have been in the form of loud rock concerts, noisy machinery, gunshots, or other loud noises. One of the most revealing tests I have ever taken was the hearing-discrimination test. I knew I had high-frequency hearing loss, so the first part of the hearing test was not a surprise. As the tones in my headphone rose in frequency, I had to strain to hear when they started and finished. My next test was hearing discrimination. The instruction sounded easy enough.

"Repeat the words that you hear me say in your headphones," the audiologist said. "Piece of cake," I thought. The words came at me one at a time. I easily repeated the words into the microphone like a trained parrot. Simple! Then I exited the soundproof booth and stood in front of the audiologist.

"Right, wrong, wrong, wrong, right, wrong, wrong, right ..." I could easily see that the wrong team was winning in this game. I also started to understand why my wife and I had such interesting conversations at home. Many of the sound-alike words that were purposefully spoken to me were misunderstood by me and repeated back as something else.

This type of hearing loss sneaks up on you. It doesn't happen suddenly. At first you may blame your poor reception on other causes. People talking, loud radios, and poor acoustics in a room often catch the blame in the beginning. But sitting across the table from someone and having breakfast is a pretty benign environment (acoustically speaking).

Working with people who have impairment to their hearing or sight requires us to change and adapt our communications skills. This may be challenging but, in the end, can be handled with just a little thought on our part.

People who have diminished hearing often become dependent on looking at the lips of the person who is speaking. People with this habit may range from those who have a long-term hearing disorder to those (like me) who have suffered the damage of rock concerts and other loud noises in their life. Typically, people look at the speaker's lips to differentiate between words, or they may ask you to repeat your statement. If you are not facing the person with the hearing difficulty, it can make it very hard for these people to understand you.

I was talking to an older patient once when he remarked how glad he was to have a male talking to him. When I inquired into his reason for the comment, he gave me some valuable information.

A female naturally has a higher-pitched voice, he said. When you have high-frequency hearing loss, you miss some of the details of the words that are spoken to you. The crux of his problem was that when he asked for a repeat of a statement, a woman would typically speak more loudly, and her voice would rise in pitch. The result was that he would have to ask for yet another repetition. He told me he had a few favorite lady nurses who had lower-pitched voices that were easier to understand.

When it comes to the vowels and consonants in the words we speak, vowels tend to be spoken in a lower-frequency range (figure 1). Consonants are spoken at a higher frequency, and often contain less energy than the vowels. The alphabet has 6 vowels (including "y") and 20 consonants, making the percentage of letters in the alphabet that are consonants about 80 percent. When the higher-frequency (and often lower-speech-power) consonants get lost, either because of hearing loss or because of a noisy environment, about 80 percent intelligibility of a verbal conversation is lost.

For a different view of this same phenomenon, write a sentence and leave out all of the vowels. Show this to someone, and chances are they will be able to easily read the sentence by mentally putting the vowels back in. Now try the reverse: write a sentence and leave out the consonants. Quite a different story!

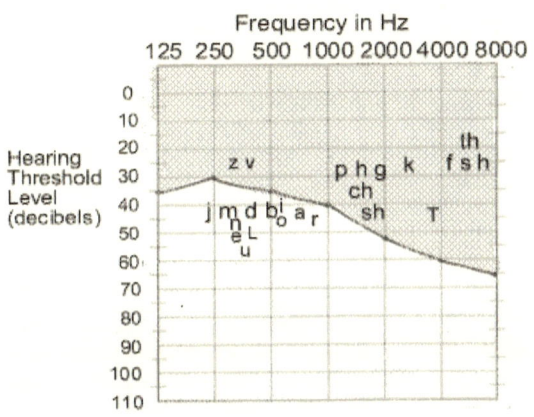

Frequency in Hz

Fig 1 Courtesy of Hound Dog Hearing, www.hdhearing.com

Another item that can interfere with the ability of someone to understand you is the presence of something in your mouth. Gum, pens, and other such objects prevent the mouth from properly forming words and distort the facial movements utilized in reading someone's lips.

Like people with hearing difficulties, people with vision impairment also need extra consideration – even when we're verbally communicating with them. You can easily understand this by just closing your eyes while in conversation with a group of people. It's common to look at

[27]

the person you are speaking to. If you can't see, how do you know if the conversation is directed to you? When speaking to a visually impaired person when there are other people around, include the person's name at the beginning of your sentence.

We all utilize many nonverbal cues in our verbal communication. You can't tell a visually impaired person that you "caught a fish this long" and hold your hands out to indicate the size of the fish. Similarly, you can't tell someone to "move over there" when they have a visual impairment, and expect them to know what direction you are referring to. Many communication cues come from the way we hold our body, move our arms, and look with our eyes. The visually impaired person can only listen to your words, tone of voice, and inflection. That being said, someone who has been visually impaired for some time has probably honed their other senses. They will be able to pick up more from your voice than people who don't suffer any impairment.

'Translation' Skills

While not recognized as an official foreign language, medical personnel often speak a language that is not understandable to most of the rest of the people in the world. Many words started off from their Latin origins and then evolved into something recognizable only to those who had acquired some type of medical certification. To complicate things further, we also have a slang version of our complicated, technical language. Unfortunately, this new language that was easily spoken between those who were certified, is unknown to those most affected by it – the patients.

As if this weren't confusing enough, we also tend to shorten things down to an abbreviation, as if just to be sure that only the chosen few know what we are talking about! We throw around acronyms like NPO and QID that affect many people but are understood by only a select group. Sometimes it is not the select group that really needs to know the meaning of what we are saying! It's important for us to be sure that our communication is understood by everyone involved, which, needless to say, includes the patient.

I once watched a new anesthesiologist talk to a patient. He asked her if she was on any anticoagulants. The blank stare from the patient showed that she did not comprehend the question. The question was repeated with a slightly raised voice. Again, the same blank look. At this point I interjected myself into the conversation. "Do you take any blood thinners," I inquired? The patient immediately looked at me and said she had taken them about a year prior but that she was taken off of them due to the bruising that occurred. Problem solved!

This is one of those situations where the correct question was posed but there was a language barrier. The doctor was correct in asking about the patient's use of anticoagulants, but the patient didn't know what he meant. Had the term "blood thinners" been substituted for "anticoagulants," there would have been no difficulty. Unfortunately, the young doctor spoke "medical," and the patient spoke "patient." Thus a barrier was in place.

We need to be sure we use terms the patient understands. Use of strict anatomical and medical wording may be the way we were trained; indeed it can be very effective to use precise medical terms with other healthcare providers. But when we speak with our patients, we need to speak laymen's language.

Of course a unique situation surrounds every patient. Some families come equipped with a nurse or other healthcare provider in the family, who can translate medical jargon. Even then, we must remain aware that the primary recipient of our communication is the patient. That means being careful that he or she understands directly what we are saying.

Unintended Communication

We have all been in situations where we are told one thing but the message we hear is distinctly different. It could be the speaker's tone of voice, the body language, or some other indicator that skews the message the speaker intended to convey.

Since we seldom have a chance to view ourselves other than in a mirror in the morning, we must be aware of the various postures and facial expressions we use that communicate meaning to those around us. Once we become aware of these, we must become conscious of them during the course of the day, to notice what we are actually telling people around us. It is very true that a picture is worth a thousand words; in this case, the picture is your posture and facial expression. The old saying that actions speak louder than words also applies here.

Over half of any message we receive comes by way of nonverbal communication: language spoken via our face and body posture. Research has shown that when someone first sees our body posture, they subconsciously try to mimic it. If we have a negative posture, then the patient will tend to adopt one also. A good, inviting, or happy posture will tend to make the person looking at us adopt a similar posture and attitude. When we smile, the people around us tend to smile as well.

Body posture can either be open or closed. Closed posture is when we place something between the person we are speaking with and ourselves. This could be as simple as folding our arms in front of us or having an object between speaker and listener. (Standing behind an over-bed table you are writing on is an example). Closed posture creates a subtle barrier to good communication. If this is the way we first interact with a patient, it sets a negative tone on the subconscious level for all future communications.

In addition to open body posture, being on the same vertical level as the patient tends to convey a message of acceptance. Standing over a patient who is lying in bed accentuates the "I-am-superior-and-you-are-inferior" feeling patients often receive from medical personnel in the course of their care. By being on the same level as a patient, we facilitate the flow of information between both parties. It can be as simple as sitting down in a chair.

Along with posture, facial expression conveys a great deal of how we feel about the person we are speaking with. Rolling your eyes, for instance, conveys annoyance, contempt, or "I've heard this line before." Establishing eye contact shows acceptance and helps to establish a feeling of trust.

Most people have experienced being the recipient or transmitter of negative signals (or both) during the course of conversations. Sometimes this was intentional, other times it was unintended and happened anyhow. Intentional or not, once this type of communication has occurred, it is difficult to remember and even more difficult to erase. When the wrong tone is set in our conversation with patients and they feel uncomfortable around us, that can result in patients withholding important information, failing to ask important questions, or doing things detrimental to their care. Our actions really do speak louder than our words!

ACTION POINTS

1._____

2._____

3._____

4._____

5._____

6._____

PLANNING

Plans are an essential part of our nursing career. Whether we are talking about a nursing care plan or our personal career plans, we need the sense of direction and purpose that a plan gives us. A plan is also indispensable to know how we are progressing. The plan is a yardstick that allows us to measure our success.

Plans are not set in stone. They should be reviewed against the goal we have set, the resources available, and the environment we work in. If a situation we are working with changes, it is appropriate to review our plan to see if it needs to be changed also.

In putting together a plan, you must gather certain items together. First, you must know what the goal is. Without an identifiable and measurable goal, you might wind up doing a lot of things without any progress in your desired direction. A good analogy would be driving your car in a circle – lots of movement, but you haven't gone anywhere. People who look very busy are usually those who are accomplishing the least. People who are familiar with goal setting and planning are typically those who place plans into action in an efficient manner, with a minimum of wasted effort.

Goals are best written down. Writing your goals allows for clarity of thought and the ability to review your goals periodically. Reviewing your goals two days, two weeks, and two months after you write them down will give you several opportunities. First is the chance to review and refresh your goals in your mind. It keeps you on track, focused, and prevents straying. Second, you can refine your goals if you look at them frequently. Maybe one goal is too broad or too grand and needs to be narrowed to allow it to be accomplished more easily. You might be able to better define your goal after looking at it several times.

General George Patton once said that "a good plan today is better than a perfect plan tomorrow." One of the greatest battlefield generals of all time, he knew the value of planning. He also knew that putting too much time into planning and holding off on implementation was a mistake.

In some circles, this is called "analysis paralysis." Over analyzing your plan (rather than engaging it) leads to inaction (paralysis). This is a favorite technique of world-class procrastinators. Trying to make your plan absolutely perfect may seem like a good thing to do, but whenever any plan meets reality, there will need to be adjustments and fine-tuning. You won't know what adjustments need to be performed if you never place your plan into action. So make a good plan, place it into action, and make adjustments as you go, as necessary.

For Patients

So what is your plan for your patient? Or more importantly, what are the goals that you and your patient have set? Goal setting should be a cooperative venture involving patient, nurse, and physician. Remember, once the goals have been indentified, then you can make the necessary plans to achieve them.

Is your goal just to get you patient out of the hospital? Is it just to shorten their stay? Or do you have a concrete goal that (hopefully) you have developed with your patient?

You may be thinking, "But I don't have time to get with my patient and decide on goals." Actually, you have been doing this type of thing for some time now. Remember discharge planning? Medicare defines discharge planning as "a process *(the plan)* used to decide what a patient needs for a smooth move *(the goal)* from one level of care to another *(goal further refined)*."

As a young nurse, I was often confused by some of the wording that people would use and the application of those words to real life. When I finally equated the word "process" with the word "plan," my understanding increased tremendously.

Goals should not be too large. Often the achievement of multiple smaller goals can lead to a sense of satisfaction while still making progress to the larger overall goal. After all, the way to eat an entire elephant is to take many small bites.

Many patient rooms have a whiteboard in view of the patient. These are often used to write down the date, nurse's name, and so on. This is an excellent place to write some of the patient's goals for that day. Items such as "Walk 100 ft." or "Use spirometer 4 times" are goals that can be accomplished in a small time frame. As a goal is accomplished, the patient can erase it off of the whiteboard. Nothing gives a sense of accomplishment quite like erasing or crossing out a goal once it has been completed.

For Personal and Professional Life

What are your goals for your life? You may find it useful to have two sets of goals in place: personal and professional. Even if these overlap, two distinct lists are advisable.

Your personal goal list might include such items as having a budget, taking steps to better your health, or goals that involve your family (spending more time with your family, attending children's sports event, etc.).

Many people routinely engage in goal setting at the start of each year. Who hasn't said they made a New Year's resolution? The problem is just that: they say it – they rarely write it down. If you have ever made a New Year's resolution, you probably recognize that most of these very well-intended resolutions fade from memory by the end of January.

Take the time to write down your goals. Put them in a place where you can see them each day. If you are the type of person who can hold yourself accountable, you might keep these to yourself. On the other hand, if you need encouragement and the help of being accountable to someone else, you might want to post your goals in a place where you and others who wish to positively support you can see them daily.

Lipstick on a bathroom mirror is not a glamorous method, but it will work. My father, who was in the Navy, often wrote to my siblings and I like this when he would be away from home for several months. This was a very effective daily reminder for all of us as to what our jobs were while he was away. Those mirrors were never cleaned until he arrived back home. A more glamorous method might be use of a magnetic whiteboard attached to the refrigerator or to some other conspicuous spot that gets looked at daily (perhaps a bathroom mirror or the dashboard of your car).

Give thought to family goals that are worked up jointly. This spreads the responsibility among several people. Maybe it is a vacation trip or a swimming pool. When several individuals buy into a project and take ownership for the results, it makes it easier to hold each other accountable. Nothing makes the job simpler than having a group of people all pulling in the same direction.

What about your professional goals? Have you given any thought to this area? The Internet has opened up many methods for nurses to enrich and improve their lives. The passage of the Patient Protection and Affordable Care Act in 2010 really opened up a new era for nurses. There will be an increased emphasis on nurse practitioners, preventative healthcare, and other areas that are ripe for the enterprising nurse to seek out.

Have you given any thought to the next 10 to 15 years of your nursing career? Where do you think you will be in that time? Knowing that life tends to take its share of sudden turns, it still helps to have a plan for your professional future. The plan can be adjusted as the many life changes occur (childbirth, divorce, eldercare issues, and so forth), but still it helps to have a plan to begin with. Your plan could involve more formal education (a master's degree or doctorate) or a change from the job setting you are in (staff nurse to case management or risk manager). If you set these plans up in advance, you more likely will be on the lookout for opportunities that help you in furthering your plan.

Don't be afraid to dream big, either. Have you ever thought about becoming the chief nursing officer of an organization? Don't think for a moment that this is out of your reach. If you set your goals and make your plan, this is more achievable. Just imagine: you, a C-level executive! The best time to think about that is now. Set your goal. Make your plans and seek out mentors to support and guide you along the way. Then start working your plan.

ACTION POINTS

1._____

2._____

3._____

4._____

5._____

6._____

LEADERSHIP

Leadership is one of those qualities that many people, mistakenly, think you must be born with. The vast majority of people don't believe you can become a leader without a background of leadership (school athletics, scouting, proper upbringing, etc.). While many youth activities do include a leadership component, and the value of such early learning cannot be denied, leadership is a learned skill.

The same as sales, marketing, or taking a blood pressure – leadership is learned. This means anyone who wishes to become better at leadership can do so. All that's necessary is seeking out the training and gaining the required knowledge. Since many people don't have the first idea of how to do this, you are on the fast track!

The first step is to realize that you are in a position to need and use leadership skills. There is no greater deterrent to learning than thinking that the time and effort you put forth will never produce results. You must be convinced that the effort you give to learning these skills will be of use to you and those around you in the near future.

Leadership skills will enable you to help patients, family, and co-workers. Knowledge of leadership skills will enhance your chance of success when you advance to positions of greater responsibility and authority. Indeed, these skills can enhance your life at work, home, and anywhere you interact with other people. Think of the many people with prior military training (who are given a constant diet of leadership training) who have gone on to become successful, high-profile leaders (presidents, secretaries of state, corporate executives, etc).

The level of leadership you achieve is not as important as how well you learn and practice your leadership skills. I read an article in *Success Magazine* where an executive moved from a small company employing 50 people to a company employing 1,000. When asked what had changed with his job, he replied, "We just added some zeros." The skill set was the same; the scale had changed.

The second step is to realize that leadership skills, much like any nursing skills, need to be studied and refreshed on a continual basis. We have mandatory continuing education for licensure renewal in just about every state for a reason – to keep you up-to-date with new information. So it is with leadership skills. We must keep up with the current thinking and new research that comes out. It is important to read (or you can listen via MP3s or CDs) about how leaders handle the various challenges that arise each day. You can then apply these same methods of leadership to your life.

What Makes a Leader

Leadership is composed of several distinctly different characteristics. An investigation into leadership components or qualities reveals many facets. Though the names may differ, these can essentially be boiled down to six primary qualities:

- Vision – The ability to see beyond the next few minutes or the next shift. Vision helps you to set goals for the future.

- Values – To know what is important, your priorities in life (integrity, professionalism, service, camaraderie).

- Communication – The capacity to listen to others and have them understand you.

- Critical Thinking – Understanding that often things are not what they seem. Looking between the lines and behind the story to seek out details that are important, then applying that knowledge to the situation.

- Empathy – To have feelings for others and understand their needs. Remember, you are leading people, not items.

- Sharing – The ability to share your vision, values, and goals for the future with others. To share the reasons and responsibility for moving the plan forward and the joy of bringing that plan to fruition. To share your skills with others and to educate them.

Leadership is also composed of different skills or methods of leadership. Compare the skills necessary for leadership during a fire (very directive, authoritarian) and those necessary for counseling someone on their future goals (goal-setting, supportive). The leadership style that is appropriate will depend on the person, their level of skill, and the situation at hand.

As people become familiar with a job and increase their skills in that job, the leader can change leadership style to one that is much more participatory. A good follower needs less direct supervision from the leader and can actually contribute input to assist the leader. The leadership style that you use will vary with the people you are leading.

Rank versus Leadership

Leadership is typically the word used when we refer to those in upper levels of management: those who are on salary, whose position starts with the word "chief," who are seen as having the power to make far-reaching decisions. In truth, these people may be policy makers or high-level managers, but true leadership is a personal skill that can be practiced at any level. Sometimes we refer to these high offices as leadership positions, though the actual practice of leadership in these positions can be a hit-or-miss phenomenon.

The civilian world rarely uses the term leadership for what is referred to as the "rank and file": those who form the base of an organization. In the medical world, we call these people "direct patient-care providers." Contrast this with the military concept of leadership that is taught to every soldier, sailor, and airman. They are expected to learn leadership skills and actively use these starting early in their training and continuing on with their career.

Leaders and Followers

Many people think that when you are a leader, you are never a follower. Nothing could be further from the truth. The CEO of a company answers to a board of directors. A general in charge of an air base has leaders above him.

In the army, a corporal may be a squad leader. In this position, he is in charge of 8 to 13 people. The corporal functions as both a leader (of his squad) and a follower (of his platoon leader). For although he is a leader, he must be an effective follower in order to integrate his unit's work with the larger levels of the organization.

Being a leader only implies that you are in a position to lead others for positive change. It is the rare person indeed who is not a leader and also a follower. Being a follower and a leader at the same time is not only common but also very normal!

So what makes a good follower? A good follower is a good team member – willing to assist the leader in accomplishment of goals the leader has shared with the group. The responsibility of followers is not just to do what they are told but to be an effective part of a team working toward a shared goal.

Can a follower have input for the leader? Absolutely. A follower should not be hesitant about bringing items to the leader's attention that will enhance progress toward the goal. A leader might not have the ability to notice every detail of a problem as the goal is engaged. Good followers either address problems as they arise themselves or bring them to the leader's attention. Leaders can be much more effective and efficient when they are leading good followers.

Being a follower allows a person to view various leadership styles and the effect they have on followers. It is through this direct observation of leadership in real time that followers become more adept at assuming their own role as leaders.

Being a simultaneous leader and follower will test your leadership skills to the max. Effective communication both up and down in the organization is a must. Critical thinking skills should be so well-honed that you are able to bring coherent thoughts to the table of your superiors, then integrate the vision and action of the larger organization into your level of leadership.

The skills you learned as a follower should still be utilized while you are in a leader situation. And when your superiors are aware of your leadership abilities, much will be expected of you as a follower. The leadership you receive will not be the directive type but more of the delegated type.

Leadership at Work

Leadership in the healthcare environment can be practiced at several different levels. Consider the nurse/patient combination.

If a nurse utilizes good leadership skills, she can effectively communicate with the patient and family a positive vision and goals for the future. She must be able to empathize with the patient in order to see and feel how the patient views the future. Are the nurse's positive vision and goals shared by the patient, or is there a conflict between how the patient and healthcare providers views things? Is education necessary to bring the patient around to the positive vision the healthcare providers have? Or do the critical thinking skills of the nurse detect an underlying problem that must be solved before the patient can focus on positive goals?

Typically, several people work with a nurse in the care of a patient. A good nurse leader can exert a positive influence on case managers, physicians, support services staff, and fellow nurses. It is important to separate the term "leader" from the term "superior." If a person in a superior position is using good leadership skills, then life is good. When the superior is not utilizing good leadership skills, then the void should be filled by anyone with the proper training and skills regardless of their position in the chain of command. True leadership, done well, seeks to enlist all people in accomplishing the goal while not necessarily being seen as an overt act. As Lao Tzu, the ancient Chinese philosophy observed: "A leader is best when people barely know he exists; when his work is done, his aim fulfilled, they will say, 'We did it ourselves.'"

Learning and practicing leadership at the patient level is essential preparation to advancing in responsibility in the healthcare field. The skills learned are not only essential to being successful as you progress up the ladder of responsibility but will make the climb much easier. A person who studies leadership will constantly seek out new opportunities to utilize current skills and learn new ones.

While the ladder you climb may include management positions, remember the words of Admiral Grace Hopper, "You manage things; you lead people." Keep your leadership (people) skills constantly honed to effect positive change in all those around you. Having good leadership and management skills will make you a better candidate for promotion.

Too many times a person with good clinical skills is promoted into a management or leadership position and is totally overwhelmed and lost. They were promoted for the wrong reason and don't have the skills to succeed in their new job. The frustration level rises until they realize that they need training (and fast) or until they resign from their promotion to go back to the security of the position they held before.

If we compare industries, the airlines don't promote flight attendants to become pilots just because they are great flight attendants. If flight attendants obtain the requisite training (flight school), they may become pilots, but it takes a completely different skill set to do the new job. Maybe we should rethink the practice of putting physicians in leadership positions in healthcare without any required training in leadership.

ACTION POINTS

1._____

2._____

3._____

4._____

5._____

6._____

CRITICAL THINKING

Critical thinking is the process of thinking beyond the obvious. It entails perceiving a self-evident situation and then going past it to seek out relevance, sound evidence, precision, clarity, accuracy, and depth.

To put this in nursing terms, let's use an example. You have a patient who is looking bad – that's the obvious. But looking closer, we ask, *why* does the patient look bad? Does his skin look different? Does his breathing appear labored? What are you defining as "looking bad" and what are the possible causes? Can you eliminate any of those causes before you call the physician?

Critical thinking is asking yourself questions about what you see. What could be causing the problem? Is there more than one causative factor? Am I missing anything? Have I ever seen this type of problem before? Do I know of someone who has? The questions should come quickly to mind. Depending on the situation, they should be answered just as quickly.

Next is the analysis stage. Through practice, we can take the answers from our questions and put them together in an analysis of the situation. If we have insufficient data, we may need to request more information to make the picture clear.

After that, we can set the priorities necessary to solve the problem at hand. It can be a patient problem, a personnel problem or something at the unit or organizational level. Regardless, the required skill set is the same. The more we think critically, the more it becomes second nature to use this process to resolve our difficulties.

Asking Questions

When an incident occurs within a hospital that is classified as a sentinel event (involving death or serious physical or psychological injury), an inquiry process is started. The process, root-cause analysis, is similar to the critical thinking process but is undertaken after the event has already transpired.

Root-cause analysis (RCA) is the process of asking question after question. Basically you want to question each answer that you come up with in order to seek out the basic, bottom-line problem. Along this journey, many items will be identified that either didn't stop the problem from occurring or compounded the original problem and let it grow until the sentinel event occurred.

Today's nurse must continually ask questions beyond the apparent. This constant inquisitiveness can uncover a multitude of factors affecting the patient. Sometimes they have been intentionally hidden (example: spousal abuse) while other times the information was withheld by accident ("oh, I forgot that I am allergic to penicillin"). We often see small signs presented to us that need to have critical thinking applied to seek out the underlying issue.

When I worked in labor and delivery, we had patients who were reluctant to open the back of their gowns for me. It greatly increases the degree of difficulty of doing an epidural when you can't see the patient's back. I would discretely ask the nurse if the patient had been subjected to any child or spousal abuse, since this type of reaction is often associated with an abuse history. On reviewing the chart, we sometimes would find a notation of such. Occasionally the nurse would then remark that she noticed the patient always covering herself up, but hadn't thought anything of it.

We must look beyond the obvious when we care for our patients. If a patient is admitted with abdominal pain and two days later, on the night shift, starts to complain of increased pain, what critical thinking should the nurse be doing? What happened to the patient during the day? Were any procedures carried out that day? Colonoscopy, barium enema, and other procedures all carry risk that could be manifested by increased pain.

Where is the pain? Is it the same pain that the patient was admitted with or is this in a different area? A physical examination of the patient, including the presence or absence of bowel sounds, may be indicated. What has the patient had to eat today? Some foods are known to cause gas pains while other foods may cause gas pains in people with specific sensitivities (lactose intolerance). What are the patient's vital signs? Have they changed recently? An increase in temperature or heart rate may herald significant changes occurring without other overt signs.

Instead of just medicating the patient, should you call the physician? If the physician on call is not the patient's normal physician, you can be sure you will get asked some of the same questions we just went over. It would be much wiser to think through all the relevant questions before making the call to the physician.

Analyzing and Synthesizing

After asking questions, the next point in the critical thinking process is to take the information you have and subject it to a rigorous analysis or review. First, run it through a quick reality check. Does it all make sense? Does all of the information agree? Lack of agreement doesn't mean that you automatically throw information out. It only means you need to verify the questionable information to determine if it is correct. The discrepancy may be pointing

[65]

you toward the problem or it could be obscuring the problem.

After analyzing the information you have, you need to synthesize a conclusion based on all of the input that you have. If it is not possible to derive a conclusion, then more information may be necessary (patient observation, lab tests, or such). It is not uncommon to develop several different scenarios from the information that you have available. Further review of the situation can guide you in deciding what other information may be necessary to derive a final conclusion.

I was performing a pre-operative evaluation of a patient one time only to be faced with two lab reports that differed significantly. Both were for the same day and drawn about two hours apart. The patient was not in any distress. I didn't have much information to analyze, but what I had was not consistent with my patient's condition. What was the problem? Further analysis of the patient information at the top of the reports revealed that only one page belonged to my patient. The other lab result belonged to someone else! It was a clerical error that had caused me to question what I saw.

Problem solved? Not so fast! The next step was to call the floor the other patient came from, determine if the other patient was still there, and tell the patient's nurse about an important lab result she needed to know about.

Setting Priorities

Priority setting is the final part of the critical thinking process. It calls for the nurse to look at the information gathered and decide if it warrants immediate action or whether it can wait until later. Part of the question that needs to be answered is what constitutes "later." The setting of priorities should include a time frame that is specific and relevant to the situation at hand.

If your hospital utilizes a hospitalist group that is in-house 24 hours a day, you may be able to safely wait an hour or two to contact the hospitalist, knowing that person is nearby and can respond quickly. If you don't have access to such a system, you might need to take into consideration the time of day. If it is 6 am, you might be able to wait for two hours until the provider makes rounds. If it is 8 pm, should you call while people are still awake and can give a quicker response? It is a very situational decision – a decision that is made more easily in the presence of good, complete, and accurate thinking.

Another component of priority setting is effectively utilizing the resources available to you. Do you have access to a rapid-response team? They may be the appropriate choice when things are happening quickly and the patient's condition is deteriorating. When you see early in the critical thinking process that things are rapidly going downhill, you can set your priorities into action while you complete the critical thinking process.

Critical thinking will set you apart as The Intelligent Nurse. It will show that you are focused, accurate, and when necessary, detail-oriented. You will be seen as the person who knows what the situation is and how to handle it.

ACTION POINTS

1._____

2._____

3._____

4._____

5._____

6._____

'NEW' NURSING SKILLS

As time progresses, the need arises to acquire new skills and materials in order to perform your job. When I was a young nurse, there were no computers to chart in. The admitting clerk in my emergency department used an IBM Selectric typewriter to input the initial information into a patient's chart. Everything else was added by hand with ink. Copies of the chart were made by carbon paper (a term that may need explanation to the younger readers out there). But time has progressed! IV bottles are now IV bags, and computers are routine. If you need to use a typewriter, good luck in even finding one.

Emotional Intelligence

"Emotional intelligence" is a term that was first coined in 1985 by Wayne Payne and later popularized by Dr. Daniel Goleman in his book *Emotional Intelligence: Why It Can Matter More than IQ*. Emotional Intelligence, often shortened down to the initials EQ, primarily refers to the following four skills:

- Recognizing your own emotions

- Managing your own emotions

- Understanding emotions in others

- Developing and maintaining good relationships

Dr. Goleman's research has shown that a high level of emotional intelligence is present in those who excel in their work despite having an IQ similar to others who don't excel. These people seem to have the skills necessary to work with others in a collaborative manner. They understand the emotional content that they bring to the table as well as the emotional drives and needs of others whom they work with.

EQ is based on the emotional skills of the individual. Complimenting those skills are other skills that include communication, self-confidence, initiative, adaptability, and conflict management. These skills are integrated to help us move forward as members of a group to achieve more than the sum of the individuals that make up the group.

Some people seem to naturally come by the various skills associated with EQ, but those who don't are not prohibited from learning. Developing the component parts of a high EQ can be accomplished several ways. Reading Dr. Goleman's books and articles is one method. Another is to do an Internet search, which will yield a number of sources (text and video) that will increase one's comprehension of the subject.

After you understand what EQ, is and develop your EQ potential you can utilize it in everyday life. Emotional intelligence is not something that is applicable only at work. Once it is learned, it can be exercised in a wide array of work, social, and family situations.

The practical application of EQ can be simply illustrated. How many times have you heard of a person who received an e-mail which they felt contained a negative tone? A person with low EQ typically types a terse reply, including a liberal dose of sarcasm and a few insults for good measure. The reply is sent at the speed of a button push. The emotion of anger sent that reply. That same emotion might have clouded the true meaning of the original e-mail. The hot-headed response might wind up being a letter of resignation!

A person with high EQ would probably read the original e-mail and reflect on its content. Is this in keeping with the established relationship between these two people? Does the message stand out as not being in line with the normal demeanor of the sender? Instead of a rapid reply dripping with acid, this message may deserve a phone call or an in-person meeting. A person with a high level of EQ would sense the emotion in that message and hold their emotions in check until the full situation is known.

The phone call may reveal that the message was not addressed correctly or was forwarded inadvertently. It might reveal that there is a situation involving higher levels at work or pressures from home that has the sender feeling flustered and frustrated.

Social Intelligence

Dr. Daniel Goleman has progressed in his research to include social intelligence. This involves the interaction between two people and how the nonverbal communication of one person can subconsciously cause a change in the thought pattern of another person. The interesting part of this process is that the subconscious mind (through the brain's amygdola) will pick up nonverbal communication faster than the conscious mind and set the tone of a conversation before the conscious mind is even aware that something is taking place.

When this subconscious awareness occurs (on the part of either party), it tends to set the tone of the entire meeting. A smile can set a pleasant tone whereas a scowl can set the tone for contention.

Emotional and social intelligence are very interesting subjects that have much to teach us all (since everyone interacts with other people), but for nurses these subjects are particularly important. I would recommend a visit to Amazon.com or your local bookstore for more information on this exciting and evolving arena.

Sales and Marketing

I can hear the cries from far and wide already. "Sales and marketing? We are nurses, professionals. We don't do

[75]

that!" Actually, we have all been doing it for years without being aware of it. Unfortunately, not being aware that we are constantly marketing works against us. We can even inadvertently engage in negative marketing!

From our earliest days (as infants and children), we have been involved in marketing and sales. You may not remember it, but when you put on a temper tantrum for your parents because you didn't want to go to sleep, you were marketing. When you protested about the food that was prepared for you that you didn't like, you were marketing. Spitting mashed peas out of your mouth is a sure-fire way to get a message across. When you dressed up before going on a date, you were definitely doing marketing. Later in life you marketed yourself to potential employers through the use of a resume. When you interviewed for your job, you were selling yourself and your professional skills as being superior to your competitors. You have a whole lifetime of marketing and sales behind you. But you didn't know that you were doing it.

The truth is that patients have a choice. Which doctor do they want to go to? What hospital will they choose? The days of having one physician, whom you see until either you or the doctor dies, is history. When the family's insurance plans change, it is not uncommon for the list of network healthcare providers to change also. This often requires choosing a new provider for your ongoing care.

The competition is out there and more than willing to welcome a new patient to their facility. Changes in provider often occur when friends talk about the care they have received and how they value their experiences. While not everyone has the same wants and needs in a healthcare provider or hospital, people will typically give high credibility to what a trusted friend has to say about their care. When that happens, it causes a ripple effect that extends much farther that we think. ("Well, I have a good friend who visited her aunt in the hospital, and she said ...")

When a patient is discharged from our healthcare facility, we seldom think of repeat business. With few exceptions (such as maternity services), we really hope that the patient will continue in a state of good health and not need our services again. We tell the patient and family to have a nice day and place them on their way out the door. We don't have to worry about them anymore – or do we?

The truth of the matter is that a vast amount of informal marketing occurs through word of mouth. Forget the billboards. Forget the TV commercials. Forget the newspaper ads. Word of mouth is truly one of the most powerful marketing techniques available. How does word-of-mouth marketing begin? It starts with a personal experience. It may by the experience of the patient or of a family member. It may be the experience of someone having an outpatient procedure or an extended hospital stay. But it always starts with a personal experience.

Word-of-mouth advertising is a two-edged sword that, once a patient leaves our facility, we have very little control over. Depending on the experience, the advertising may be positive or negative. It may be based on one or two impressions, but those impressions represent the person's experience in a nutshell. Positive or negative, we can't change those impressions once a patient or family member leaves. This brings to mind the old saying that "you don't have a second chance to make a first impression."

[78]

Unfortunately, negative word-of-mouth marketing tends to spread faster and farther than its positive sibling. When a negative story is retold, it tends to become even more negative over time. Much like the fisherman's tale of the fish that got away, when a bad experience has taken place, it tends to grow and become worse the more times it is talked about.

Marketing experts say that a person who has a positive experience will tell three people about it while a person with a negative experience will tell ten. Three versus ten – the odds are not in our favor!

The advent of modern technology has added a whole new dynamic to the word-of-mouth marketing system. Facebook, Twitter, and other forms of instant and mass communications can spread a story (good or bad) around the globe at slightly less than the speed of light. And instead of talking to one or two people at a time, a person has a potential audience of thousands! Unfortunately, emphasis is still on the negative healthcare experiences, because people expect that good or great care should be the norm (and they are right).

We indeed live in an age where every action we take has a consequence. A seemingly trivial comment you make can have very strong and negative repercussions. Simple, random acts of kindness can also return to you and your organization thousands of times over. We must become aware of the impact of our actions and words on the organization. Those who think the patient only has one place to receive medical care are mistaken. Even in a county with one hospital, there is usually an alternate place to receive medical care 20 or 30 miles down the road. With good transportation, this means a trip of 30 to 40 minutes. This is not an insurmountable trip when the alternative is a facility that you think gives bad medical service.

Medicare keeps voluminous statistics derived from patient questionnaires. One such survey is known as the Hospital Consumer Assessment of Healthcare Provider and Systems (HCAHPS). This survey, which is not restricted to Medicare recipients, allows an apple-to-apple comparison of healthcare facilities and the providers within them.

Data published in 2010 reveals some very interesting information. A correlation study between the different areas reported in the HCAHPS was performed. It was found that the section on nursing communications has the highest positive correlation with 7 of the 9 areas reported. Indeed, in the section on how you would rate the hospital, nursing had its highest positive correlation.

Nurses, through their actions and interactions, have a profound effect on the perception of healthcare in general and their hospital and nursing in particular. We can ill afford to squander even one opportunity to provide world-class service.

Many nurses are probably appalled at the thought of being expected to become salespeople. I know of some nurses who sell various products at work to other employees, but they would never dream of selling to the patients. Yet sales skills are exactly what is needed to get the patients to "buy" better health habits for the long term.

Sales today are based on the establishment of a relationship between the purchaser and the seller. If a good relationship is not created, you have one person telling the other what to do. How would you like to go the store and have the clerk tell you, "Buy these pants"? Most likely you

[81]

would turn around and leave the store. There was no relationship built up at all. The salesperson is after a sale that will never occur.

But what if the sales clerk approached you with a smile, greeted you, and made a flattering comment about the jewelry you were wearing? The seeds of a relationship have just been sown. Usually what follows is some idle chit-chat about the color of the jewelry or the design of an item of clothing. The astute salesperson is listening to you (verbally and nonverbally) as your words and postures tell her about yourself, your tastes, and your needs.

At this point, you feel that the salesperson has an interest in you as a person, that you are not just another sale to be written up. So the salesperson moves on to the second part of the sale: painting the future picture in your mind.

After taking you to a section of clothing, the clerk may select a dress with colors to match the jewelry you talked about. She may then tell you how the item suits you or how well it compliments your style (assuming it actually does – sincerity is essential in effective selling!)

[82]

What the clerk is now doing is painting a picture that you can visualize in your mind about your future if you purchase that item of clothing. If the picture is appealing, before you know it, you have a magnificent image of how great you're going to look if you buy that article.

That picture is painted with a color called "benefits for you." It is not colored with features of the clothing (50 percent rayon, "one of the last we have in pink") but with the benefits you will receive if you make the purchase (less hassle with the laundry, making a knockout impression at the party). Sales professionals know that you want to know WIIFM (What's in It for Me). This is where the picture of benefits becomes critical to making the sale.

How can we apply this scenario of successful selling to our profession of nursing? The first thing any good salesperson does is determine what they have that they want to sell. So what do we have on the sales rack today?

- Wellness and health

- Better behavior

- Compliance with medication and treatments

These are broad categories, but you can customize them once you begin a relationship with the patient and learn of their unique needs.

At a glance, these three sales rack items seem pretty boring and dull. The Intelligent Nurse will search out the ways necessary to paint a picture that has the patient ready and willing to do the things required to make that future picture come true.

As in the clothing store analogy, we first must build a relationship with the patient. In the case of certain elderly and all pediatric patients, we may need to build a relationship with key family members as well.

Does building a nurse/patient relationship sound difficult? It's easier than it sounds. What about the admission assessment that was done when the patient arrived in the hospital? If you are not the person who admitted the patient, take a minute to read that and learn about the individual. Working or retired; married, divorced, or widowed – there is a vast amount of information available that should not be ignored. When you walk into the patient's room, what do you see? Are there magazines or books in the room? If so, what are they about? What is on the TV? How about polite conversation? If you make a comment about the weather, the patient might respond with a comment about gardening, outdoor sports, playing with grandchildren, or something else that will give you a clue about their values and interests. These are all items that will help you form the relationship necessary to sell the patient on better health.

Now it is onto the second step of selling: painting the future picture. Make sure that it is an upbeat picture. People like positive things, so be optimistic. You could paint a picture of how the family will look at the funeral since the patient didn't take her blood pressure medicine, but that hardly qualifies as a future picture that many patients will work with!

Paint the picture with a view to how much more the patient will enjoy going to football games as he loses weight and can navigate his way in the stadium more easily. Paint a picture of how many more holidays the patient can enjoy with the grandchildren as her blood pressure is kept in

[85]

control by regularly taking her medication. A diabetic may enjoy your providing a picture of being taken off insulin injections if they lose weight and stay on a good diet. You must show the patient the benefits they will enjoy from the effort they put forth. There has to be a payback for the patient, the WIIFM factor.

It will sometimes require imagination and resourcefulness to paint the correct picture. Don't be afraid to enlist the help of family and friends to learn about the patient and what they like. While personally people may be quiet about themselves and their accomplishments, family members are usually very proud of what the patient has done in the past and will toot his horn for him.

Continue to use and build upon the relationship that started the first time you met the patient. By learning to market and sell better health, you will help your patients heal – not only in the hospital but long after they return home, as their new, more positive lifestyle restores them to greater happiness and vitality.

ACTION POINTS

1. _____

2. _____

3. _____

4. _____

5. _____

6. _____

CONCLUSIONS

The skills we were all taught in nursing school will serve to make us safe, basic, entry-level nurses. Notice the words "safe," "basic," and "entry." That essentially means that we won't kill anyone we come in contact with for the first 24 hours. Okay, maybe the first 12 hours!

To become The Intelligent Nurse of the 21st Century, we must learn other skills that will set us apart from the great majority of nurses. Remember, each of us is but one part of approximately 3 million nurses – 3 million highly trusted individuals who have a personal impact on every patient they come into contact with.

For the Patient

Patients and their families expect to be treated effectively and efficiently. If they are seen by a provider, taken care of, and sent home in the same or better shape than they arrived in, most people won't complain, but they won't be impressed either. We are in a profession that takes pride in providing excellent care of our patients. Should we be satisfied that the patient views her encounter with the healthcare system as a neutral event? Why shouldn't we strive to provide a positive experience that the patient will want to tell others about? Is there a reason to only treat the presenting disease and ignore the total person – a person who will be in our company but for a short time and then have only occasional exposure to sellers of better health?

For the Organization

Most organizations exist as the mere sum of their parts. If your organization has five parts, then the sum of that organization can only be five. But what if the parts were not typical parts but supercharged? What if that same organization, with five parts, was not just the sum of those parts but much more?

Organizations with supercharged parts will be organizations that survive and flourish in the ever-changing field of healthcare. They will adapt to the new requirements and still deliver on their promise to their consumers, the patients. These organizations will be agile enough to adapt while other organizations get stuck on the old ways of doing things that no longer work.

The Intelligent Nurse is a supercharged nurse, a driving force for innovation who can keep her organization safely afloat amid the shifting tides of change. Hospitals operate under complex reimbursement systems, and reimbursement rates will decline for average and poor organizations in the future. The resulting cuts can cause a downward spiral that is extremely hard to recover from. Protect your organization from extinction by making it superior!

The Intelligent Nurse is aware of such outside forces and the impact they can have on every person within the organization. Leadership from below can result in ideas being put forth that will help keep the organization on the cutting edge of quality care. Such leadership almost has to come from below, since the upper-level leaders are usually occupied with problems from above. Their tunnel vision and singular focus frequently prevent them from seeing the

[91]

simple solutions that can have such a positive impact on patients. In the end, the mighty are lead by the least of them.

For the Individual

Some of the ideas presented in this book seem new and strange to many nurses. Indeed, these are items that have seldom been brought forward. We have often been content to bask in the glow of what we already know, thinking life is good and we know all we need to understand. But just as we had to learn many new ideas and concepts when we went to nursing school, time has changed the field we work in, and we must continue to learn, or become obsolete.

The healthcare system of yesterday is gone forever. It won't come back, no matter how hard we might wish for it. Having been involved with this profession since 1971 (when I started nursing school), I can attest that nursing of the past bears faint resemblance to nursing today. If I had stayed with only what I had been taught, I would be a dinosaur by now.

Times change, and I changed also. Increased knowledge gives us the ability to accept increased responsibility. If you look up the quotation "Knowledge is power," you will find it attributed to several different people. It is not just the philosophy of one person, this idea that we empower ourselves with increased comprehension – it is the idea of many of the greatest people who have ever lived.

We must continue to adapt in order to provide the quality healthcare we so often talk about. It is one thing to talk the talk. We must now, more than ever, walk the walk.

For the Profession

As nurses, we need to move forward in the nursing care of the patient, to take the bold steps necessary to finally become the formidable force in healthcare that we like to talk about. While each day is a new dawn for us individually, and a new dawn is here for our profession today.

As this manuscript is being written (summer and fall 2010), many changes are happening to healthcare in general that are opening doors like never before for nurses. In

[93]

October of this year, a report was released called *The Future of Nursing: Leading Change, Advancing Health.* Prepared by the Committee on the Robert Wood Johnson Foundation Initiative on the Future of Nursing, at the Institute of Medicine, the report paints a new picture for our future as nurses. The principal findings are as follows:

1. Nurses should practice to the full extent of their education and training.

2. Nurses should achieve higher levels of education and training through an improved education system that promotes seamless academic progression.

3. Nurses should be full partners, with physicians and other health professionals, in redesigning healthcare in the United States.

4. Effective workforce planning and policy-making require better data collection and an

improved information infrastructure.

IOM (Institute of Medicine). 2011. *The Future of Nursing: Leading Change, Advancing Health*. Washington, DC: The National Academies Press.

While the report is almost 600 pages long, it is only a vision for the future written by 30 people. It will take the action of 3 million nurses to change this vision into a reality. We must step up and take the individual steps necessary to put these findings into action. If we don't, then when we are asked why nursing didn't change like people said was possible, we only have to go as far as the nearest mirror to find the reason. Let us remember those powerful words by Goethe, "Knowing is not enough; we must apply. Willing is not enough; we must do."

ACTION POINTS

1._____

2._____

3._____

4._____

5._____

6._____

ABOUT THE AUTHOR

Long ago, a young man saw the progress in the field now known as emergency medicine. Advanced first-aid was giving way to medical treatment in the pre-hospital setting. That teenager thought that one day in the future, nurses would be providing that early, critical treatment. So Donald Wood entered the nursing program at a junior college right after graduating from high school. That was 1971.

Since graduation from Florida Junior College at Jacksonville in 1973, Donald has been providing direct patient care in a variety of settings. He graduated from nurse anesthesia school in 1977. Through the many years Donald has always remained true to the fact that, no matter what he does, he is a nurse.

To say that he is part of the nursing family is an understatement. His wife, Debbie, is a nurse as is his daughter. Three sisters-in-law are nurses and his brother-in-law's wife is a nurse.

Along the way, Donald served as a decorated member of the U.S. Air Force Reserve. His duties included clinical anesthesia administration, disaster relief coordination, and teaching in a leadership school for five years. He was awarded the Air Force Achievement Medal in 2004. He left military service with the rank of Lieutenant Colonel.

Donald lives with his wife in North Central Florida and continues to administer anesthesia, while working as a healthcare consultant and writing with the endeavor to improve nursing for patients, the profession and the individual nurse.

For more information on The Intelligent Nurse and Donald Wood ARNP, visit:

DonaldWood.com

TheIntelligentNurse.com

 Visit our blog at:

Blog.TheIntelligentNurse.com

www.ingramcontent.com/pod-product-compliance
Lightning Source LLC
Chambersburg PA
CBHW022111170526
45157CB00004B/1576